IKIGAI

UNLEASHING THE JAPANESE SECRET TO ATTAIN LONG LIFE, FIND HAPPINESS AND FULFILLMENT

DIYA GREG

Made with ♥ on the Notion Press Platform
www.notionpress.com

Contents

Contents

Title Page

IKIGAI

Unleashing the Japanese secret to attain long life, find happiness and fulfillment

Diya Greg

CHAPTER ONE

Definition of Ikigai and its historical development in Japan

The Japanese concept of ikigai relates to having a reason to get up in the morning or having a purpose for existence

It is a notion that describes the point at when one's passions, skills, the needs of the world, and the possibility of financial reward all converge.

Okinawa, a Japanese island with one of the world's greatest life expectancies, is where the concept of ikigai was first developed.

Researchers and professionals in the area of longevity have studied and respected the Okinawan people because of their purposeful and connected way of life.

The concept of ikigai in Japanese culture refers to a way of living that prioritizes one's emotional, intellectual, and social health in equal measure.

It exists over the lifespan and manifests itself in many facets of living, including professional endeavors, recreational pursuits, interpersonal connections, and the cultivation of one's own identity.

People all across the globe have turned to the notion of ikigai in recent years as a method to improve their quality of life and achieve their full potential in their personal and professional endeavors.

There is no better moment than now to refocus our efforts, and properly plan out our dreams and objectives for the future, while we continue living and enjoying life and trying to maintain those well-intentioned but high New Year's resolutions.

Despite the fact that the "new year, new me" motto is encouraging, maybe there is a more effective strategy for embracing all that life has to offer if the only thing motivating us to improve is a new number on the calendar.

Japanese philosophy called ikigai has long been linked to the country's legendary longevity.

Taking its name from the Japanese terms for "life," "iki," and "value," "gai," ikigai is the pursuit of living with meaning.

In other words, your ikigai is the driving force behind your day-to-day activities.

Finally, let's define ikigai.

The term "ikigai" has its roots in ancient Japan, namely the Heian era (794 to 1185).

Clinical psychologist and passionate specialist in the ikigai development, Akihiro Hasegawa produced a study paper in 2001 where he stated that the term "gai" derives from the word "kai" which translates to "shell" in Japanese.

Shells were highly prized throughout the Heian era, and this period's economic prosperity left an indelible mark on the word.

Similar meanings may be found in the Japanese phrases hatarakigai (働きがい), "labor value," and yarigai g aru (やり甲斐がある), "it's worth accomplishing"

Having an ikigai is what pulls you out of bed in the morning and keeps you working hard.

Discovering your gai, or life's meaning, is essential.

Looking at the ikigai Venn diagram, which depicts the overlap of the four key qualities—what you are excellent at, what the world needs, what you can be paid for, and of course, what you love—is the greatest way to properly absorb the underlying idea of ikigai.

To reduce it to its barest essentials, we might say that ikigai exists at the intersection of these two ideas.

CHAPTER TWO

Why Ikigai is crutial and vital

Researchers and theorists in the fields of sociology, science, and journalism have come to some fascinating conclusions on the significance and use of this phenomena.

It has been theorized that if you find your ikigai, you will live a longer, more purposeful life.

Kyotango, a village in Kyoto, is proud to have three times as many people over the age of 100 than the rest of Japan, so in September 2017, the popular Japanese TV show Takeshi no katei no igaku collaborated with a group of scientists to undertake study there.

Seven folks in their late 90s and early 100s were followed about from morning 'till dawn as they had blood tests and other health check-ups on the show's premise of discovering the parallels between these old happy people and themselves.

DHEA, a steroid hormone generated by the adrenal glands, is thought by many to be the magical "longevity hormone," and the researchers discovered that all seven persons had extraordinarily high levels of it.

However, when the show followed these individuals about, they discovered that they all had a passion for a daily activity.

People of all ages were out and about on any given day; one lady in her late 90s was spotted spending many hours a day crafting traditional Japanese masks; another guy painted; while another went fishing.

The show stated that engaging in a pastime you like might enhance your levels of the young hormone DHEA, which in turn can contribute to a longer and happier life; however, the link between the two has not been scientifically verified.

How vital it is in finding your purpose

Many factors highlight the significance of identifying one's life's raison d'être and pursuing it with fervor:

1 It gives you a feeling of direction and satisfaction in life when you discover and pursue your true calling.

The process enlightens you to the significance of your actions and decisions in the grand scheme of things.

Having a strong sense of why you're doing something may give you the drive to go out there and give it a shot, and it can also encourage others to do the same.

What's more, it may motivate you to think outside the box and persevere even when things go tough.

Three, it boosts happiness because when you're following your passion and living your purpose, you're more likely to feel good feelings like contentment, fulfillment, and appreciation.

As a result, this has the potential to boost health and quality of life in general.

Passion for one's work is correlated with increased productivity, concentration, and dedication, all of which contribute to better overall performance.

Better results in your personal and professional life may result from this.

Finding one's calling and following it increases one's odds of making a positive difference in the world (point #5).

Everyone around you, and even the world at large, may reap rewards from your efforts and decisions.

The positive effects of adopting an attitude of "Ikigai"

The Ikigai philosophy may help you find success and pleasure in these ways:

First, you'll acquire clarity and concentration on what really matters to you since the process of discovering your Ikigai will reveal this.

As a result, you may better link your beliefs, skills, and aspirations with your life's direction.

Living your life in accordance with your Ikigai gives you a feeling of direction and significance.

If you have a meaningful life, you won't have to force yourself out of bed in the mornings, and you'll be more driven to follow your dreams and have a great impact on the world.

Third, your well-being will improve if you follow your Ikigai and devote your time and energy to the things that make you happy and fulfilled.

In addition to making you feel good, this will also make you feel more accomplished and less stressed, anxious, and depressed.

Fourth, you'll have better interactions with people if you follow your Ikigai every day.

It's possible that your increased genuineness, kindness, and positivity can help you forge more fulfilling bonds with others.

5. Enhanced inventiveness and originality This is a byproduct of living in accordance with your Ikigai.

If you are driven by your passion and sense of purpose, you are more likely to generate original ideas and find effective approaches to problems.

Ikigai is a Japanese concept that refers to the driving force behind one's activities and the means by which one might have a beneficial effect on the world.

What part of the world do people engage in ikigai?

Okinawa, a southern island of Japan, has one of the highest rates of centenarians per capita in the world.

It's no surprise that Okinawa is a center of ikigai thought.

The island's active population of non-retiring, purpose-driven people is what connects them to other long-living communities like Sardinia, Italy, and Icaria, Greece, despite the island's favorable climate, nutritious food, and low stress levels.

There are some of the world's longest-lived individuals in Okinawa.

In his book Blue Zones: Lessons on Living Longer from the People Who've Lived the Longest, published in 2010, author Dan Buettner analyzed regions of the globe with the longest-living populations (including Okinawa).

What he found was that ikigai, or having a "purpose in life," was a powerful unifying thread even though various cultures use different words for it.

If you're excellent at what you do and it brings you joy, you've discovered your ikigai.

Hector Garcia, author of many books on the topic (including the recent Ikigai: The Secret to a Long and Happy Life in English), disagrees that ikigai should be associated only with the elderly.

In fact, its popularity among young people, both within and outside of Japan, is at an all-time high right now.

For example: "We noticed that the timing of the term 'ikigai' is one of the keys to the success of the book's release."

He claims that the time has come, "particularly among younger generations yearning for greater purpose in their life," for it to receive widespread acceptance.

Locating your hobbies and passions

Discovering your Ikigai and leading a meaningful life begins with understanding what you care about.

A few suggestions may help you zero in on your true interests and passions:

To start, focus on the things that make you happy:

Take note of the things you like doing that bring you joy and satisfaction.

These topics are likely to spark your interest and enthusiasm.

Consider what you aspired to be when you were a kid, the things you wanted to accomplish.

Some insight into your deepest interests and motivations may be gleaned from these.

Third, branch out and try new things; doing so may lead to the discovery of previously unknown hobbies.

Participate in an activity that interests you by joining a club, taking a class, or volunteering.

Think about what you hold dear and what you believe in; this brings us to our fourth point: reflect on your values and beliefs.

Your deepest beliefs and ideals will likely inform the pursuits that mean the most to you.

Five, solicit the opinions of others: often those closest to us may shed light on our true interests and passions.

To find out what your loved ones and coworkers believe you're excellent at and what you seem to like doing most, you may ask them directly.

Keep in mind that it takes time and introspection to discover what it is that really drives you.

Trust your gut and your curiosity to lead you to the things that make your heart sing.

CHAPTER THREE

Knowing your Ikigai

Garcia claims in his book that learning about the ikigai philosophy has influenced how he approaches each day.

I've streamlined my daily routine so that I spend some time each day on self-care before attending to the needs of others.

In other words, he gives top priority to his most important responsibilities.

Green tea, 15 minutes of gentle yoga, and an hour of writing are my typical morning routines.

Before going, I focused on my health and on one of the things that gives my life ikigai: writing.

Despite its professional connotations, ikigai is not necessarily about making money.

Ikigai may take the form of a very satisfying activity, the joy of raising a family, or the ability to strive toward the realization of a lifelong dream.

Admitting your competence and talents

Finding your Ikigai and making the most of your life requires first realizing what you're good at.

Aware of your abilities? Here are some pointers:

Be aware of your strengths and inherent abilities:

Consider the activities that don't need much mental or physical exertion on your part.

These abilities are probably those you were born with.

Second, focus on your best qualities:

Think on your strengths, both in your work and personal life.

Your greatest advantages will presumably lie in these areas.

Third, take stock of your accomplishments, both large and minor.

How did you learn to do those things?

Fourth, solicit the opinions of others:

Find out what your loved ones and coworkers value most about you by inquiring about your abilities and talents.

Other people's viewpoints and insights might help you see your own strengths in a new light.

5. Participate in assessments or personality tests There are a plethora of assessments and personality tests available online.

Results from these assessments might provide light on your unique blend of characteristics.

Understand that it takes time and introspection to become aware of your own unique set of strengths and abilities.

Don't be afraid to branch out and try something new; just remember to believe your gut when it tells you something is a good fit.

You may have a richer, more meaningful life if you take stock of and put to use the gifts God has given you.

Ikigai Consists of Four Main Parts

The essence of your ikigai is at the crossroads of many different aspects of your existence.

The Japanese notion of ikigai relies heavily on these four pillars:

1. Your mission in life should take into account both your own motivations and the external demands of the world.

One's ikigai is tied to a higher purpose.

The ikigai principle suggests that at least a quarter of what makes life worth living is finding ways to improve the lives of others.

Inspiration: Investing in one's own growth is a demanding but ultimately worthwhile endeavor.

Finding your own ikigai, or the pleasure you get from doing what you were here on this earth to do, is just as important as doing your part for the greater good if you want to uncover the meaning of life.

You should figure out what it is that you like doing the most, and then devote the rest of your life to doing it.

Profession: Ikigai implies making a genuine impact in the world via your work.

One essential part of developing a complete ikigai is discovering a calling in your work that you like.

Try to choose a job that not only helps others but also interests you and makes you happy.

4. Talent: If you know what you're innately excellent at, you've nailed down another crucial component of your ikigai.

Inquire about the skills you currently have and those you desire to improve upon, especially among the younger generations.

If you want to live a happy and long life, it's possible that you should spend each day doing something that brings you joy, is easy for you to accomplish, and benefits others.

Seeing the world's problems and the ways in which you may help

Discovering your Ikigai and leading a successful life requires you to have a firm grasp of the world's needs and the unique value you can bring to the table.

Read on for advice on figuring out what the world really needs and how you can help it:

First, you'll need to pinpoint the issues plaguing society:

Try to find places where society is struggling, as with poverty, inequality, or the environment.

Answering these tests may help you better understand the wants and requirements of the global community.

secondly, think about how your viewpoint differs from others:

Reflect on how your unique set of experiences, abilities, and perspectives may help solve social problems.

As an individual, you have a fresh viewpoint that might lead you to solutions.

Next, investigate prospects: find groups or organizations that are tackling social issues that resonate with your beliefs and interests.

One way to help is to donate your time or seek employment with one of these groups.

Considering how your interests and abilities might be used to resolving social issues is an excellent topic for introspection (see also point #4).

If you have a knack for photography, for instance, you may utilize your talents to educate others about environmental problems.

If you want to know how you may better contribute to society, you should ask for advice from people you know and trust, such as friends, family, and coworkers.

Other people may be able to help you see your own strengths and how you might put them to use.

Keep in mind that it takes time and introspection to figure out what the world needs and how you can help.

Don't be afraid to go out and try something new; instead, let your gut tell you where your efforts will have the most effect.

You may give your life greater meaning and purpose by learning about the world's needs and how you might meet those needs.

CHAPTER FOUR

Guide to locating your Ikigai

You can regain your sense of direction and concentration if you've lost sight of your ikigai.

If you're having trouble moving forward because change is challenging, Garcia advises trying something new. This may be anything from picking up a new pastime to making some extra cash at a side job.

In his 2017 book, The Little Book of Ikigai: The Essential Japanese Way to Finding Your Purpose in Life, Tokyo-based neuroscientist, writer, and broadcaster Ken Mogi argues that "you are a cleaner of the famous Shinkansen bullet train, the mother of a newborn child, or a Michelin-starred sushi chef";

You have succeeded in locating your ikigai if what you do is pleasurable and satisfactory to you. I would say a big congrats to you.

Ikigai may take the form of a pastime, the joy of raising a family, or the ability to strive toward the realization of a lifelong dream.

As Garcia puts it, "develop knowledge of the present situation of your life" if you're having trouble making ends meet.

Begin by making a list of the top 10 activities you've engaged in this week.

After making a list, you may evaluate whether or not the items on it are helping you live a more fulfilling life.

The process of subdivision may be broken down into four questions:

How much do I like doing it?

To what extent does the world have a need for it?

Ask yourself:

- Am I any good at this?

Is this anything that would earn me money?

If you can't make a living doing it, ask yourself whether the alternative is worth it in terms of sustaining your ikigai.

Don't worry if you're having problems committing since studies have shown that ikigai, like a person's choice in music, clothing, and ideas, can alter and evolve with age.

It's never too late to start enjoying life; the retirees in Takeshi no katei no igaku all found new passions by the time the book ended.

Maybe this year you should shift your attention from short-term goals to the long-term goal of discovering your ikigai.

Discovering the place where your interests, abilities, and opportunities converge is the key to thriving.

The essence of the Ikigai concept is finding the intersection of your interests, abilities, and opportunities to have a positive impact on the world.

Find your niche with these helpful hints:

Then, figure out what drives you.

Take some time to ponder and record the things that actually motivate you.

Interests might range from specific interests like a pastime or a cause to general ones like a way of life.

Second, acknowledge your abilities:

It's important to recognize your strengths and interests.

These characteristics probably represent your skills and abilities.

Think about the issues that others are experiencing and how you may help solve those problems, and then ask yourself what the world needs.

Which problems or movements do you find yourself most invested in?

4. Be on the lookout for promising prospects:

Investigate many options until you find one that fits your interests, skills, and aspiration to make a difference in the world.

There are a wide variety of options, from helping out in your community to studying and working in an area that interests you.

To find your optimal performance zone, you need to explore and iterate.

As you gain knowledge about yourself and the world, be adaptable in your approach.

Finding your niche is not a destination, but rather a journey of self-improvement.

The key to a happy and productive life is finding a way to combine your interests, skills, and experiences.

Creating routines and behaviors that support your Ikigai

Developing routines and practices that serve your Ikigai is crucial if you want to live a life that matters.

In order to better assist your Ikigai, here are some suggestions for establishing routines and habits:

Establish a daily routine:

Whether it's writing, exercising, or meditating, begin your day with practices that support your Ikigai.

Doing so will establish a good mood for the day and help you concentrate on your goals.

Goal-setting is the second step:

Create a plan of action for achieving your objectives that is in line with your Ikigai.

Maintaining your drive and concentration in this way is crucial.

You should prioritize your interests and hobbies.

Set aside time every week to pursue hobbies that really inspire you, whether they be music, art, or outdoor recreation.

Make time for exercise, rest, and a balanced food as part of your routine for self-care.

These actions keep you motivated and on track with your objectives.

Fifth, put yourself in the company of individuals who will encourage and inspire you.

Having this kind of group around you may be a great source of inspiration and drive.

It's important to keep in mind that it takes time and work to form new habits and routines.

The key is to take things slowly and reward yourself for even the smallest achievements.

You may lead a happier, more meaningful life by establishing routines and habits that serve your Ikigai.

CHAPTER FIVE

Pursuing your Ikigai and discovering significance and happiness along the way

Pursuing your Ikigai in a way that brings you purpose and happiness is crucial to having a full and satisfying life.

How to get fulfillment while chasing your Ikigai:

1) Have fun with it!

Keep in mind that the pursuit of your Ikigai is a process, not an endpoint.

Accept the inevitable ups and downs of the road and treasure the lessons you'll pick up along the way.

Make an effort to appreciate the gifts of life as they are bestowed upon you.

Doing so helps in maintaining an optimistic outlook and a concentration on the positive aspects of life.

Third, savor the victories along the road, whether they be the completion of a project or the reaching of a significant milestone.

You'll be able to keep your enthusiasm up and your mind on the task at hand.

Take some time to think on how far you've come and what you've learnt.

Being aware of your progress and the next actions you need to do is a great way to keep moving forward.

5. Take pleasure in the journey, not just the destination: Remember that the journey itself is as rewarding as the destination when it comes to finding your Ikigai.

Learn to take pleasure in the journey itself, as well as the experiences and relationships you have along the way.

Keep in mind that the pursuit of your Ikigai will take time and effort, but will ultimately be rewarding.

Keeping a cheerful attitude, appreciating progress, and taking pleasure in the journey all contribute to a richer, more meaningful existence.

Finding ways to use your Ikigai in your day-to-day activity

To achieve happiness and success in life, it is crucial to integrate your Ikigai into all aspects of your existence.

Here are some ways to make your Ikigai a part of your daily life:

Get your values in line with your Ikigai:

Find your Ikigai and make it a reflection of your particular ideals.

That's a great way to start living a life that's really your own.

Make it your mission to find work that allows you to put your Ikigai into practice by actively seeking out and seizing chances that do just that.

Finding significance and value in your job is facilitated by this.

You should prioritize your interests and hobbies.

Set aside time every week to pursue hobbies that really inspire you, whether they be music, art, or outdoor recreation.

Uncover ways to make a positive impact on your neighborhood by volunteering or joining local organizations.

By doing so, you will find yourself among others who share your interests and values.

Five, prioritize connections that support your Ikigai by hanging out with like-minded individuals.

Having this kind of group around you may be a great source of inspiration and drive.

Keep in mind that you must put in time and effort to make your Ikigai a part of your business and personal life.

The key is to take things slowly and reward yourself for even the smallest achievements.

Living a life that is both meaningful and satisfying may be achieved by bringing your career and personal pursuits into harmony with your Ikigai.

Striking a good note in everything that you do

Strive for internal and external consistency if you want to have a happy and healthy existence.

If you're struggling to maintain equilibrium in your life, consider these suggestions.

One must first learn to prioritize their time:

Figure out what's most important to you and focus on it.

This aids in maintaining concentration on the essentials and warding off fatigue.

Limit your time and energy expenditures to prevent yourself from being overburdened.

This keeps you from getting so caught up in chasing your Ikigai that you forget to take care of yourself.

Third, take care of yourself by giving yourself a break and doing things you like, like exercising, getting adequate sleep, and eating well.

These actions keep you motivated and on track with your objectives.

Create a network of individuals who believe in you and will be there for you when you need them most while you follow your Ikigai.

5. Interrupt your routine at regular intervals to rest, rejuvenate, and assess your performance.

You'll be able to keep your enthusiasm up and your mind on the task at hand.

Just keep in mind that it takes consistent work and reassessment to achieve a state of equilibrium in your efforts.

If you want to make sure you have a long and happy life, you need to be adaptable and ready to make adjustments as necessary.

By maintaining a sense of equilibrium and harmony in your life's activities, you may enjoy more happiness and success without jeopardizing your health.

CHAPTER SIX

Make a positive impact in your world by sharing your ikigai with others

Your Ikigai is the driving force that motivates you to make a difference in the world and to share that passion with others.

One of the keys to a happy, satisfying existence is to help others and to leave a good mark on the world via your Ikigai.

The following are suggestions for effectively communicating your Ikigai to others.

The first step is to tell others about what you care about; this may be done via social media, public speaking, or any other means of expression.

You may find other people who share your interests and establish a strong network of friends and allies.

Discover ways to give back to your community through volunteering, making charitable donations, or mentoring those less fortunate.

You can make a difference in the world and strengthen your feeling of purpose by doing this.

Third, provide an example for people to follow by leading an interesting and rewarding life yourself.

Inspiring people in this way may lead to a domino effect of good change.

Fourth, work with others to make a good impact in your town or field. Find others who share your beliefs and interests.

When you do this, you may combine forces and make a bigger difference than you could on your own.

5. Show compassion and understanding to people, no matter their views or origins.

You may strengthen your connections with others and leave a lasting mark on the world by doing this.

It's important to keep in mind that spreading your Ikigai and making a difference in the world are never-ending processes that need your whole attention and energy.

The key is to take things slowly and reward yourself for even the smallest achievements.

You may have a more meaningful life and make a difference in the world by helping others discover and pursue their Ikigai.

With your Ikiga, you will develop and change throughout time

Maintaining a dynamic relationship with your Ikigai is crucial if you want to lead a life that matters.

If you want your Ikigai to develop and change over time, consider the following:

In a first step, be adaptable and willing to try new things that bring you closer to your Ikigai.

This allows you to maintain flexibility and progress.

Second, evaluate whether or not your present activities continue to be in line with your Ikigai on a frequent basis.

This aids in maintaining focus and preventing you from straying from your goal.

Third, make some new targets: Make some new targets that fit in with your Ikigai and push you to develop and improve.

This aids in your never-ending quest for self-improvement and enlightenment.

4 - Continually expand your knowledge and expertise in areas that relate to your Ikigai via study and experience.

This keeps you interested in and committed to your mission.

The fifth step is to actively seek input from people who share your beliefs and interests.

You may gain wisdom and insight from the experiences of others by doing so.

Keep in mind that nurturing and developing your Ikigai over time calls for consistent work and commitment.

The key is to take things slowly and reward yourself for even the smallest achievements.

By nurturing and expanding your Ikigai, you may lead a more meaningful life and make a difference in the world.

Motivation to make each day count

We all want to find ways to make our lives count, to have an impact.

This is a process, not an endpoint, and it will need your constant attention and energy.

These words of inspiration are meant to help you find greater purpose and happiness in your life.

1) Do what makes you happy; pay attention to your inner voice and focus on developing the skills that will help you achieve your goals.

Have confidence in yourself and trust your gut.

Value your individuality and embrace what makes you special.

Recognize your own strengths and put them to good use in the world.

Avoid negative self-talk by focusing on your own progress rather than that of others.

Don't sit around and wait for chances to present themselves; instead, get out and make them.

This keeps you interested in and committed to your mission.

Put yourself in the company of upbeat, encouraging individuals who share your interests and ideals; this will do wonders for your mood and outlook.

The result is a group of people that have your back and cheer you on.

Count your blessings and appreciate the good things in your life rather than dwelling on the bad.

A more optimistic outlook and more gratitude for the positives in life are the results.

Just keep in mind that it's a long, winding road to a life you love and find purpose in.

Be willing to learn and develop, but never close yourself off to the possibility of experiencing joy or success.

Making a difference and leaving a legacy behind is possible via leading a life of purpose and fulfillment.

The End

Printed by Libri Plureos GmbH in Hamburg,
Germany

9 798889 868255